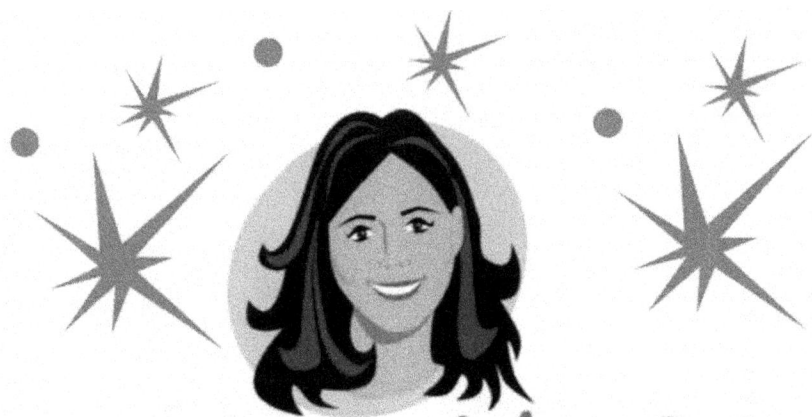

The
Conscious Living Guide™
with *Christine Agro*

10 Ways to
Naturally Avoid
Colds and Flu
(and what to do when they come knocking)

Christine Agro

Liability/Warranty:

The author has made every attempt to provide the reader with accurate information. This information is presented for information purposes only. The author makes no claims that using this information will guarantee the reader or the reader's family health and wellness. Readers are advised to check with their family doctors before using information provided in this book. The discussion of websites, procedures and other information contained in this book are current as of the date of publication. The author shall not be liable for any loss or damage incurred in the process of following the information presented in this book.

The Conscious Living Guide ™
www.theconsciouslivingguide.com
christine@theconsciouslivingguide.com

DEDICATION

To the natural healers in my life:
Grandma Mamie, Nan and Dad. Your natural approach to health and wellness seeped into my soul and fuels my passion for naturopathic healing.

ACKNOWLEDGEMENTS

To everyone who supports me, knowingly, unknowingly, consciously, unconsciously; and to everyone who has helped me learn, heal and grow – Thank you!

A SPECIAL THANK YOU TO
Chuck Agro, Caidin Agro, Trudy and Bill Viscardo,
Gertrude Rieker, Mamie Viscardo
Farida Sharan, Lauren Skye,
Grace Morgan, Divya Chandra, Diane Caldwell, Maria Fergosi,
Grace Coddington, Nan Bush and Bruce Weber

Table of Contents

Our Dependence on Doctors Keeps Us…Dependent. 1

    What Contributes to Colds and Flus? 2

    When Should We Be Most Vigilant? 2

An Ounce of Prevention is Worth a Pound of Cure. 3

Preventative Natural Healing Support 5

Inside the Body 5

Your Goal 5

    Heal Thyself goes hand and hand with Know Thyself. 6

    What Natural Healing is Not 7

        It's Not Magic 7

        It's Not Isolated 8

        It's Not A Quick Fix 8

        It Doesn't Mean You Won't Get Sick 8

        It's Your Body, It's Your Responsibility 8

        Healing Crisis 9

        Use Common Sense and Trust Your Own Instincts 10

        Understand Your Fear. 10

    Preventative Natural Healing Tools 11

    Tool #1: Diet 11

    Tool # 2: Foot Reflexology 12

    Tool #3: Probiotics 13

    Tool #4: Vitamin D 14

    Tool #5: Apple Cider Vinegar 17

    Tool #6: Liquid Chlorophyll 18

    Tool #7: Bee Propolis 19

    Tool #8: Essential Oils 22

        Diffusing 23

        Topical 23

        Essential Oils to Support Health and Wellness: 24

        Basil, Sweet (Ocimum basilicum): 25

        Cistus (Cistus Ladanifer/Labadanum/Rock Rose): 25

        Clove (Syzygium aromaticum): 25

        Eucalyptus (Eucalyptus globulus): 25

        Geranium (Pelagronium graveolens): 25

        Lemon (Citrus limon): 25

        Marjoram (Origanum majorana): 25

        Tea Tree Oil (Melaleuca Alterniforia): 25

Neroli (Citrus aurantium): 25
Peppermint (Menta piperita): 25
Ravemsara (Ravensara aromatica): 25
Rosemary (Rosmarinus officinalis CT 1,8 cineol): 25
Rosewood (Aniba rosaeodora): 25
Thyme (Thymus vulgaris CT linalol): 25
Tool #9: Raw Juices 26
Apple: (not bottled apple juice) 27
Orange (not from a carton) 27
Carrot 27
Spinach 27
Tool #10: Colloidal Silver Spray 28
Tool # 11 Homeopathy 29
The Outside World? Out of Your Control? 32
WASH YOUR HANDS! 32
Extra Support – Natural Hand Cleaner 32
The Dreaded Note From The School Nurse OR Bob is Sick as a Dog and
Working Right Next to You! 34
Condition Specific 35
Conjunctivitis/Pink-Eye 35
Colloidal Silver Spray: 35
Castor Oil 35
Sore Throat/Strep Throat 36
Tea Tree Oil 36
Hydrogen Peroxide 36
Apple Cider Vinegar/Hot Water/Lemon/Pinch of Cayenne/Honey . 36
Oil Pulling 37
Cold/Flu 37
Homeopathic Remedy 37
Epsom Salt Bath 38
Turmeric Milk 40
Essential Oil 41
Cough 41
Apple Cider Vinegar Drink 41
Oil Pulling 41
Herbal Support 41
Homeopathic Remedy 42
Liquid Chlorophyll 42

Diarrhea/Constipation 43
Just In Case 45
Wrapping It Up 46
Notes: 47
References 48
About Christine Agro 50

Our Dependence on Doctors Keeps Us...Dependent.

I wrote the first edition of this book in 2009 when the word 'pandemic' was being used in almost every other sentence. The 'pandemic' at hand was the H1N1 virus.

I wanted to offer not only a calming voice, but also strategies to help people stay healthy, avoid the flu and be able to support themselves, should they get sick.

Fast forward to today, it's 2013 and we are experiencing, according to the media, the worst flu outbreak in years.

I was at a store the other day and I overheard a woman talking on her cell phone. She was talking to someone who apparently had the flu and her advice was to 'get to the doctor and get some tamiflu.'

I did a quick check of Tamiflu and not only is it expensive, $100 for 10 tablets, there is a list of possible side-effects among which are nausea, vomiting and diarrhea. Isn't that what you take it to help with?

I'm not opposed to western medicine but I do feel that we are too reliant on it. We have replaced our body's ability to self-heal with prescriptions for pills that do the work for us, but in the doing of the work, we get farther and farther removed from our innate ability to heal.
Self-healing can take time. It isn't a 'quick-fix' like most of what western medicine offers. It does require that we connect with and understand our bodies and that we understand the process of healing.

When we use natural remedies, we are working with the body, to help support it and in offering this support, we slowly rebuild our body's natural ability to heal.

In Naturopathic medicine, prevention is the starting place. It is our goal to offer the body all that it needs to stay healthy and in balance.

The more we honor our body and work with it, the stronger our natural healing responses become if or when we do get sick.

What Contributes to Colds and Flus?

We have created a perfect storm that lends itself to disease. Over time we have been systematically depleting our natural ability to defend against disease through the foods we eat, the stress we experience and the medications we take that suppress the body's ability to defend itself. We are depleting our bacteria and virus fighting Vitamin D because of concerns about the sun and we continue to move farther and farther away from embracing our own intuition and knowingness.

When Should We Be Most Vigilant?

As we approach the Fall, the days get shorter and we have less access to the sun. We start to retreat indoors increasing our exposure to each other and to each others germs.

Throughout the Winter, again, due to our close proximity, less daylight and even the stress of the holidays, our immunity can become less than optimal.

As Spring arrives, our system goes through another shift and our immune system can be challenged.

In the Summer mostly head colds arise due to fluctuations in temperature. We go from the extreme heat to the frigid air-conditioning of stores and movie theaters and then back out to the heat; or we fall asleep with a window open and an unexpected cool night breeze stresses our system and voila, we have a cold.

You may also notice that you or your child have a habit of getting sick at a certain time of year other than these

So you can see, there is no singular time that we are more inclined to get sick. That's why prevention is the best way to support yourself. I think rather than seeing your efforts as 'avoiding getting sick' it would be more helpful and even productive to see your efforts as 'what you can do to stay healthy.'

By incorporating the suggestions in this guide, you can support your health and wellness and that of your family and experience less colds and less flu. You will benefit by learning how to boost your own health and wellness, naturally and simply, empower yourself and learn more about your own body, what it needs and how giving it support provides a worthy return on investment.

With our children, it is not only important but empowering to help them tap into their natural healing abilities. While they are young, they are still open and connected to their inherent healing ability. Help them retain it. Teach them that the answers lie within and help them see that the medical community is there to support rather than hold the view that the medical community knows more, or has more power.

Advisory: since no two people are identical, this information provides a guide. This guide does not guarantee health or wellness. We are each responsible for our own choices. Please consult your doctor or your child's pediatrician if you question how something will interact with a condition you have been diagnosed with or with medications you are taking.

An Ounce of Prevention is Worth a Pound of Cure.

So said Benjamin Franklin and, boy, was he right. Don't wait until you're coming down with something. Start to build your health and wellness now.

I hope that the easy to follow suggestions in this book will help to keep you and your family cold-and flu-free now and forever.

Remember, you hold the key to your own health and wellness. It isn't something that rests outside of you. Our bodies come equipped with the natural ability to heal, but we need to support our bodies so that this ability can function. Western medicine overrides this natural ability and western diet undermines this ability.

In natural healing we focus on supporting the body's natural ability to self-regulate and self-heal. When we offer resources that enable the body to maintain its natural balance and assist in fighting off disease, we strengthen our natural ability to heal. If on the other hand we use Western medicine's approach of addressing symptoms with synthetic (man-made) products, we override the natural ability of the body, systematically reinforce a message that the body cannot heal itself and we become more susceptible to dis-ease.

Our Western diet is also a factor in our health and wellness. We are the only culture which focuses on nutrients rather than food.[1] As with so many things in our culture that pertain to health and wellness, we have applied the science of the mind in understanding how our body uses food and have broken this process down into vitamins, minerals, and amino acids. In using the science of the mind we eliminate the holistic perspective of how foods work within the body.

Science does the same thing when it tries to determine if an herb or natural supplement "works." Science studies in isolation and looks at one specific element, herb, vitamin, mineral or natural remedy to pronounce whether it is effective or not. The body doesn't work that way, nor do the things that support the health and wellness of our systems. We work holistically. Herbs work holistically. Food works holistically. This is why I do my best to support the body with whole and natural sources whenever possible.

---

[1] Michael Pollan, _In Defense of Food_ (New York: Penguin Group 2008) pg 19 - 32

Preventative Natural Healing Support

Inside the Body

Where health and wellness are concerned, the most important function of the body rests in the eliminative channels. The body has five primary channels – the bowel, the kidneys, the lymph, the blood and the skin. Each eliminative channel helps to process toxins out of the body and the channels work to support each other. If one channel is out of balance or taxed, the others work harder to offset the imbalance. The more out of balance the system becomes, the greater the potential for disease to set in.

Iridologists (use of the markings, colors and textures of the iris to assess the strengths and weaknesses of the body) will tell you that the bowel is the key. Of the five main eliminative channels, toxicity in the bowel has the ability to impact the entire body because from an iridology stand point, the bowel is reflexive (connected through neuro pathways) to every area of the body.

In my iridology studies, everything from heart problems to seizures have been corrected by addressing the toxic build-up in the bowel. When it comes to our immune system, a healthy bowel equals a healthy immune system. A sluggish bowel equals a sluggish immune system.

Since keeping the bowel healthy is a key to *staying* healthy, your first three health and wellness tools are connected to not only keeping the bowel functioning optimally, but also keeping the other eliminative channels working at their best.

Your Goal

Your goal is to keep the body functioning in a healthy and balanced way. The more you are able to do this, the greater your chances are of keeping colds and flu at bay and the greater your chance is of stopping a cold or flu before it takes hold.

To keep the body functioning optimally there are number of very simple things you can do that will greatly enhance the healthy balance of your body.

It's not difficult; in fact some of the things are common sense. It does however, require that you take responsibility for your own health and wellness and despite how it sounds; many of us are just not that good at doing this. We move through our lives unconsciously and only pay attention to our body when it 'yells' loud enough for us to listen. This is another key element of natural healing: the willingness to be healthy and stay healthy needs to be a conscious choice and one that is front and center in our daily lives. It requires that we understand, or at least begin to acknowledge all of the components that support or detract from our health and wellness.

Heal Thyself goes hand and hand with Know Thyself.

Although 'Heal thyself' comes from a proverb found in Luke 4:23 and refers to critics taunting Jesus to perform the same miracles for himself that he performed for others, it has taken on a meaning in Natural Healing that refers to our ability to 'heal ourselves'.

When I was doing my Naturopathic and Herbal studies at The School of Natural Medicine, the program was rooted in experiential studies. Our learning was based on personally exploring every remedy, treatment, diet and herb that we might recommend to others and to undertake a dedicated course of healing ourselves.

What I have learned over the years is that in order to heal ourselves, we have to know ourselves, or at least be interested in learning more about ourselves. This is where personal power comes from; it comes from being curious about who we are and what we are capable of doing and being. It comes from being willing and open to exploring that which we don't know. It comes from digging deeper into that which we do know, always questioning information and absolutes.

Just as so many dichotomies are coming to the forefront of our awareness (Republican/Democratic ideologies; within the Roman Cahtolic Church) the difference between the Western approach to medicine and the Natural approach to medicine illuminate yet another dichotomy. In Western medicine we are asked to hand over our power, to accept what the medical community has to say and to believe that they are more knowledgeable then we are. In Natural Healing we are asked to take responsibility for our own health and wellness, to understand how our body works and to support it holistically. This doesn't exclude the use of Western medicine, but it does exclude the belief that doctors know more.

To heal thyself, we need to know thyself.

What Natural Healing is Not

Before we get started, there are a few things I want you to remember about Natural Healing: It's not magic, it doesn't work in isolation, it's not a quick fix, it doesn't preclude getting sick, you are responsible, use common sense and understand your own fears.

Natural healing is powerful, but it requires that we think and live differently. We can't use Natural Healing as we would Western Medicine and expect it to work, and we shouldn't assign attributes to Natural Healing that are untrue.

It's Not Magic

Natural healing is not magical. It may seem like it sometimes, especially when you are witness to your body self-healing; but it is not magical. When you treat your body holistically and support it naturally, you are tapping into a powerful system, just like a car that works optimally when it is provided high quality oil and fuel and tuned-up regularly.

It's Not Isolated

Natural Healing is not isolated – meaning, we aren't looking for a single remedy, we are looking at the body as a whole and providing the support it needs to stay healthy, that could be a combination of nutritional, dietary and physical support.

It's Not A Quick Fix

Unlike western medicine, which often offers a quick fix, natural healing can take time as it works to support the body's natural ability to heal. Consider the process of a cut healing; it takes time for the body to knit the skin back together, however, the healthier you are, the quicker the healing can occur. So our goal is to stay healthy! The 'quick-fix' although seemingly immediate does nothing to build your own immune system; in fact, it can detract from it by suppressing and masking your symptoms. Then, rather than taking the time to get well, you push yourself further, believing you are well, which further impacts your own health and wellness.

It Doesn't Mean You Won't Get Sick

For some reason people tend to think that natural healing means they should never get sick. I often hear people say 'oh, I tried that, it doesn't work. I still got sick.' Natural healing, natural support, natural remedies don't prevent you from ever getting sick, but they do help you create a strong, healthy, naturally responsive immune system. If you are supporting yourself naturally, if or when you do get sick, you may still feel awful, but your body will be better equipped to heal itself.

It's Your Body, It's Your Responsibility

I can't stress this enough: your body, your responsibility. We have gotten so far away from taking responsibility for ourselves. We want others to tell us what to do, how to do it and to do it for us and even worse we want to blame others for whatever doesn't go 'right'. Natural Healing requires that you empower yourself to be responsible for your own health and wellness.

8

If you want more information about something, research it. If you try something and you don't like the reaction before you toss it out as a remedy consider this: is this your body just responding to suddenly being supported in this way? There are many remedies that I use that cause diarrhea when I first use them. I see this as my body cleaning out what needs to be cleaned out, I don't stop the remedy. If my reaction is strong, I may stop until my body resets and then start at a lesser dose. But I don't stop before I even get started. But I know many people who stop right there. They are either fearful of the experience, or inconvenienced by it, so they stop.

Healing Crisis

We cannot become healthy without healing those things that contribute to our un-health. Our bodies will experience what is known as a 'healing crisis' when we start to use natural supports. Now, 'healing crisis' sounds much more dramatic than it actually is. A 'healing crisis' is simply the body's way of clearing, purging, cleaning and resetting itself and the crisis might include diarrhea, fatigue, nausea and in some cases vomiting. But here's the good news, if you go slow with your process, you can oftentimes mitigate or completely avoid any healing crisis. And unlike 'side-effects' to medications, once you move through a 'healing crisis' your body is stronger and healthier as it is part of the healing process.

Natural Healing requires that we get in touch with our own body and learn to listen to it. In a way it is a very different process from working with Western Medicine, but in others it really isn't. Sometimes it takes trial and error, but if you think about, that's actually not that different from Western Medicine. How many times have you or someone you've known gone to the Doctor, ben prescribed a medicine, only to have it not work or to have an adverse reaction to it? When you let your Doctor know, he either prescribes something else or changes your dosage. You don't look at this as 'failure' though, you take it as part of the process. Natural Healing has that same process of testing to see what works and what doesn't.

Use Common Sense and Trust Your Own Instincts

If something doesn't resonate with you, then don't do it. If you aren't sure about something, get more information. If you wonder how or why something works or doesn't work; do some research.

Understand Your Fear

Sometimes we have fear and it is warrant, but often we have fear and it is a signal that we are hitting up against energy and information that limits us. A great example is when I had my son. I was already a Naturopath and a Master Herbalist. I used Natural Healing with myself, my animals, family and clients. But when my son was born, I suddenly found myself fearful of using remedies with him. The weight of being responsible for him, somehow made me lose my certainty. It took me about a month to get my bearings and clear that fear. Be conscious of your fear and be honest about it. Where does it come from and what is it telling you. Mine was coming from social programming that we all deal with, that programming that says 'we can't heal ourselves.'

Preventative Natural Healing Tools

Tool #1: Diet

When supporting the body, diet is of course important. Dairy products such as cow's milk, cheese, ice cream and cream cheese as well as too much bread, pasta and meat can cause mucus build up and inflammation in the bowel which then affects other areas of the body.

Eating a diet that is rich in fruits, vegetables, nuts and seeds will greatly support your health and wellness.

Caffeine, soft drinks and processed juices (more sugar than juice usually) do nothing to support your health, and everything to contribute to deficiencies.

Consider this fascinating piece of information from one of my favorite books, *Nutritional Herbology* by Mark Pedersen: Iron, which is important to our immune system, is regulated by absorption within the body. Tannic acids, egg yolks, milk, cheese, carbonated soft drinks, and even aspirin form insoluble precipitates with iron and can lower the iron absorption rate. Coffee and tea for example reduce iron absorption by 50%. [2]
And this is just one of many important connections between food, nutrition and wellness.

As we approach cold and flu season, cut down on excesses, eat foods in moderation and be conscious of your intake of the foods listed above.

As Michael Pollan says in *In Defense of Food*: *"Eat food. Not too much. Mostly plants"*.[3]

---

[2] Mark Pederson, <u>*Nutritional Herbology*</u>, A Reference Guide to Herbs, Revised and Expanded Edition Wendell W. Whitman Company, 1998 p 20.
[3] Pollan, p 1

Tool # 2: Foot Reflexology

Reflexology is the practice of massaging areas of the feet to help promote healing in other areas of the body. It is believed (and I concur) that all areas of the body are represented on the soles of the feet.

If you take your thumb and press around your feet, you're likely to find areas that are sore. This soreness is an indication that areas of your body are out of balance.

Doing regular reflexology work on yourself or your child will help to keep your body working effectively. The reflexology work helps to keep the energy flowing through your body.
In acute situations (immediate rather than long-term) such as the on-set of a stuffy or runny nose, the flu, fever and coughs, foot reflexology does wonders to reduce or altogether eliminate the congestion in the bowel and set you on a quick road to recovery.

It is interesting because once you become accustomed to your feet or your child's feet, you will be able to feel the difference when you or they are not well or something is coming on. In Foot Reflexology, the area of the bowel, which can be found just above the heel on the sole of the foot, will feel spongy or sometimes harder in certain areas or you may find what feels like crystals as you massage the area. The more you work out this energy, the clearer the digestion and the bowel will become. You can often times fend off a bug taking hold, or clear it up more quickly by using foot reflexology.

For a Reflexology Foot Chart visit:
Wallet Foot Charts are $3.00
8 ½ x 11 charts are $11.00

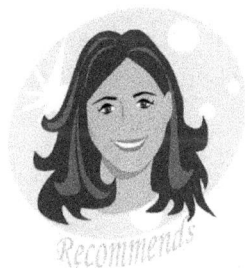

http://www.reflexologyseminarsofny.org/index/mn35010/Store

12

Tool #3: Probiotics

Probiotics are a dietary supplement that help support the positive bacteria that populate the bowel and also support the digestive process. Probiotics offer a great way to keep the bowel working well in general. It is available as a dietary supplement (most often associated with lactobacillus, although that is just one strain) and can also be found in foods such as yoghurt and miso.

Of note is a 2005 study in Sweden, in which "a group of employees who were given the probiotic Lactobacillus reuteri missed less work due to respiratory or gastrointestinal illness than did employees who were not given the probiotic."[4]

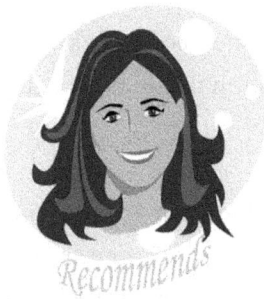

For adults: I personally take Megaflora by MegaFood.
It is free of Gluten, Dairy, Soy, Pesticides & Herbicides. Does Not Contain Corn and is a Validated Nutrition.
You can find it in the Health Store (refrigerated) or on-line.

Recommends

For children: I highly recommend Nature's Way Primadophlus for Children in the powdered form. It can be mixed into any liquid. Find this at the Health Store (refrigerated) or on-line. (May contain a minimal residual amount of dairy or soy protein.)
For kids I recommend the powdered form over the chewable form because the body doesn't need to exert extra energy to break down and process the powder. It dissolves and is more readily absorbed by the body.

---

[4]"What exactly are probiotics? What health benefits do they offer?" <u>Consumer Health</u>, Mayo Clinic, (http://www.mayoclinic.com/health/probiotics/AN00389)

Tool #4: Vitamin D

Vitamin D is essential to our natural immunity. The body uses Vitamin D (which is actually considered a hormone) to create proteins that function as antimicrobial peptides. These antimicrobial peptides breakdown and kill bacteria and viruses relatively quickly.

"Scientists at the Centre for Disease Control and Prevention in Atlanta have suggested the reason we are more likely to get colds and flu in the winter is because that's the time it's hard to get enough Vitamin D."[5]

In 2008, The American Academy of Pediatrics increased the recommended daily dosage of Vitamin D for children from 200 to 400 units. Other researches feel this is still conservative and an amount up to 2000 units can be added daily.

At the core of the Vitamin D deficiency is our retreat from the sun. Our bodies cannot make Vitamin D without outside help. It is a vitamin that the body makes when it is exposed to the sun. Ten – twenty minutes of sunlight exposure on just arms and legs daily will provide approximately 3000 units even during the winter months. Amazingly, twenty minutes of *full* body exposure will assist the body in creating 20,000 units of Vitamin D within 48 hours of exposure. (exact units depend on the intensity of the UVB in the sun, skin color, and location.)

-----

[5] "FEELING PEAKY? YOU NEED MORE SUN! Good Health: As Research Shows Vitamin D Is Vital to Health, There's Only One Answer," <u>The Daily Mail (London, England)</u> 3 Apr. 2007: 51, <u>Questia</u>, 1 Aug. 2009 <http://www.questia.com/PM.qst?a=o&d=5020097012>.

Additionally, unlike supplementation, when the body naturally creates Vitamin D, there is no risk of Vitamin D toxicity. The body naturally regulates the Vitamin D production and converts any excess. According to Sunshine Vitamin (an organization that advocates natural Vitamin D through regular, non-burning exposure to the sun) while overexposure to sunlight carries risk, no research has shown that regular, non-burning exposure to UV light poses a significant risk of skin damage.

What about Vitamin D through food sources? You will see in this list that although foods can and do provide sources for Vitamin D the amount provided isn't substantial.

Source IUs per Serving[6]

- 360 IUs: 3.5 ounces Salmon cooked
- 200 IUs: 3 ounces canned Tuna
- 250 IUs: 1.75 ounces Sardines (canned in oil, drained),
- 98 IUs: 1 Cup Milk, Vitamin D–fortified
- 60 IUs: Margarine, fortified, 1 tblsp.

If you are going to take a Vitamin D supplement, you should first get a blood test to confirm supplementation is necessary. It is possible to overdose on Vitamin D supplements – remember, naturally created Vitamin D is self-regulated by our body, but supplementation is not. Once you determine the need for supplementation, from my research, the best option is a Vitamin D gel cap that contains fish liver oil. This source will provide Vitamin D3. If you choose to supplement Vitamin D, it can take six to seven weeks for Vitamin D levels to peak in the body, so keep this in mind as you begin to supplement.

---

[6] "Dietary Supplement Fact Sheet: Vitamin D", Office of Dietary Supplements, Dec. 11, 2008, National Institute of Health, July 10, 2009, (http://ods.od.nih.gov/factsheets/vitamind.asp#h3)

Do not exceed:

　　2000 units daily for adults
　　1000 units daily for infants
　　2000 units daily for children

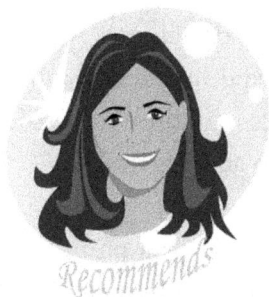

Recommends

For Adults: MegaFood Vitamin D3 1000 IU or 2000 IU

For Kids: Kid's n Us Vitamin D3 400 IU Can be found in Health Stores and on-line.

Both kid and adult versions are whole food nutrients.

Tool #5: Apple Cider Vinegar

Raw Apple Cider Vinegar offers wonderful natural healing support. It helps reduce inflammation, balances pH, acts as a natural digestive enzyme and helps boost the immune system. I wouldn't be without it as cold and flu season approaches. Taking it regularly will give you an excellent preventative. Some recommend rinsing the mouth after drinking ACV to protect the enamel on the teeth. Others have suggested drinking through a straw to by-pass the teeth. I find taking it diluted tends to address any issues, but if you have concern, the two options above help to address those.

I recommend Raw Organic Unfiltered Apple Cider Vinegar over pasteurized versions. The Raw ACV has the mother, which is an active enzyme. Pasteurized versions don't offer the same natural healing support.

ACV offers both preventative and healing support (see the Condition Specific section below for specific uses).

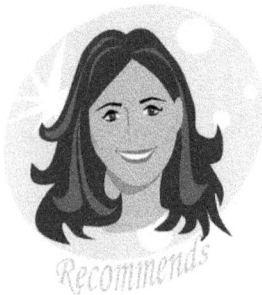

Brand: Bragg's or Eden's brand
Where to find: Health Store
2 tsps in 16 oz of water sipped throughout the day
In winter heat it up – it makes a nice hot drink.

Recommends

Tool #6: Liquid Chlorophyll

Liquid Chlorophyll is expressed from Alfalfa, which is one of the most vitamin and mineral complete herbs. Liquid chlorophyll helps to pull toxins out of your system. It removes them from bones, joints, cells, tissue, lymph and blood. It is a whole food supplement, which means it cannot be over-consumed. It is also said to function like hemoglobin and helps to generate red blood cells.

Not too long ago I had an annoying dry cough that would just not go away. After living with it for over a month and losing a lot of sleep, I remembered Liquid Chlorophyll. I began drinking 1 teaspoon in an 8 oz glass of water 3 x a day and by the second day I was no longer coughing.

Liquid Chlorophyll offers both preventative and healing support.

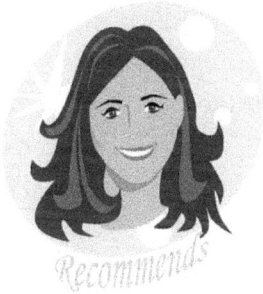

Brand: World Organics Unflavored Liquid Chlorophyll (uses organic alfalfa). I prefer the unflavored to the mint flavored.
Where to find: Health Store / on-line
Recommended dosage per Label: 1 tablespoon in one 8 ounce glass of water daily; may take any where from 1 teaspoon to 1 tablespoon in one 8 ounce glass of water to up to three glasses a day.
Caution: Liquid Chlorophyll stains. It will turn stool green and in some cases may cause constipation if enough water is not consumed.

Tool #7: Bee Propolis

When it comes to preventative health and wellness, Bee Propolis is one of the most effective and supportive natural remedies available to us today.

Propolis is considered an herb because it changes little from its material state. Propolis is comprised of resins which bees collect from tree buds and bark. When tested, the propolis is almost identical to the original resins seeping from the trees, which is why it is classified as an herb. Bees use it to fortify the hive; not only using it to seal up minute holes, but also using it to prevent disease, parasites and bacteria from entering the hive.

Bee Propolis has been used since ancient times as both a topical and internal healing agent. There is record of it being used by the Egyptians, the Greeks and the Romans, by the Incas in the 11th century and by the French in the 18th and 19th centuries.

Topically it can be used to heal burns, cuts, wounds and warts. It is an effective anti-fungal and anti-microbial agent and has been effective in eliminating MRSA (antibiotic resistant bacteria). Most of the information about the effectiveness of Bee Propolis is anecdotal amassed over thousands of years of use. Today though there are a handful of laboratory and clinical studies that have examined both the anti-microbial and anti-fungal potential of Propolis.

In 2004 a study was published by an Israeli research group in the Archives of Pediatric and Adolescent Medicine. The group studied 'the effectiveness of a syrup containing Echinacea, Propolis and Vitamin C in preventing respiratory tract infections in children.'[7] The study included 430 children ages one to five years old with one group receiving the herbal remedy and the

---

[7] C. Leigh Broadhurst, Ph.D., Jack Challem Editor, *Basic Health Publications User's Guide to Propolis, Royal Jelly, Honey and Bee Pollen: Learn How to use "Bee Food" to Enhance Your Health and Immunity.* Basic Health Publications, Inc., 2005, Kindle Version, Loc 303.

other receiving a placebo. Of the children who took the herbal remedy, there were 55% less instances of respiratory tract infections and if these children did get sick, it was for a shorter period of time.

Additional studies have been done in the Netherlands, Romania and Poland all showing that Propolis acts as a preventative for respiratory tract infections and greatly reduces the recovery time in contracted cases, when used in combination with antibiotics.

Caution: Both adults and kids can take Bee Propolis, but if you have bee allergies then you may be severely allergic to Bee Propolis; additionally if you are uncertain, the same concerns are valid. If you don't know if you have a bee allergy, you can avoid Propolis altogether, or you can do a test by taking a small amount and observing your reaction. Logic would tell us, do it when others are around so you can get help if you need it. As always, if you are uncertain about any type of remedy, consult your doctor before using it.

Usage

Topically you can mix Propolis with raw honey to place on open wounds. Interestingly, antibiotic topical ointments can be overused just as oral antibotics and lead to antibiotic resistant skin bacteria. It is wise to find alternative ways of avoiding infections.

Internally, the recommend dosage is 500 mg daily for prevention. I advise taking it two weeks on and two weeks off or five days on and two days off particularly during high cold and flu season. By taking a break it lets your body's own immune system reset and strengthen, rather than being consistently fortified. If you feel yourself coming down with something, take with 1000 mg for a few days and see if you can ward whatever it is off.

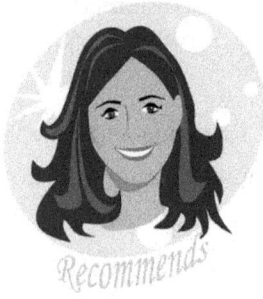

Books on the use of Bee Products

If you are interested in learning more about Bee Propolis and the many benefits of all bee products, I recommend you read '*Basic Health Publications User's Guide to Propolis, Royal Jelly, Honey and Bee Pollen: Learn How to use "Bee Food" to Enhance Your Health and Immunity*' by C. Leigh Broadhurst, Ph.D.

Brand: Y.S. Organic Bee Farm: Propolis Raw-Unprocessed 1000 MG (tablet = 500 MG of Propolis extract)

Tool #8: Essential Oils

For use with:

- Newborns – no oils unless diffused and no oils containing menthol or camphor
- Infants – do not use any oil which contains menthol or camphor (up to 30 months)
- Toddlers - OK
- Pre-Schoolers - OK
- Kids – OK
- Adults – Ok

Therapeutic grade essential oils are different from synthetic fragrances. Synthetics are man-made scents often found in body care products and room fresheners that offer no therapeutic value. Additionally they may contain chemical by-products that cause them to detract from your health and wellness, rather than benefit you as true essential oils will do.

My husband knows that I love lavender and I love Epsom Salt baths, so he was very thoughtful and brought home a box of Lavender scented Epsom Salt. As soon as it hit the water, I knew it was synthetic fragrance – the more you work with essential oils, the more you can easily pick out synthetics. They just don't have the same purity and vibration of true essential oils.

Therapeutic essential oils are distilled essences from plant material, which do offer therapeutic value. When you use therapeutic grade essential oils, you provide your body with excellent support in combating bacteria and viruses. Oils have been used throughout the ages in everything from healing to skin care and they offer a range of supporting properties: antimicrobial, antibiotic, antiviral, calming and antifungal, to name but a few.

There are many ways to work with essential oils, but for the purpose of this book I'm going to cover just two – diffusing and topical application.

Diffusing is wonderful not only because it supports the health and wellness of the body, but your home or office will smell lovely too.

There are a number of ways to diffuse oils but the best, in my opinion, is with a nebulizer.
The nebulizer uses a cold high pressure process to break apart the oil and disperse it into the air; other processes use heat, which can augment the nature of the oils.

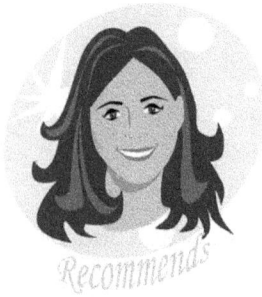

There are a number of nebulizers on the market and I recommend that you check out www.diffuserworld.com – lots of options to choose from; however, I love the Aroma-Ace. I LOVE this nebulizer.

Topical application is also very beneficial. I have used topical application of essential oils to soothe a cough, reduce a fever, stop a sore throat, relax, and relieve a stiff neck.

Stiff Neck

> *Caidin woke up one morning with a stiff neck and couldn't move. He was both in pain and frightened. I grabbed a few essential oils, massaged them into his neck and held him. Within in an hour he was up and running around.*

Strep Throat

> *A few years ago I went home to help my Mom, right after my dad had passed away. She had day surgery at a local hospital and I spent the day at the hospital with her. The next day my throat started to get sore and I unfortunately did not bring any of my natural remedies with me and my mom had no apple cider vinegar or liquid chlorophyll. By the next morning I had strep throat. Seeing as how I was with my senior mom and my five-year-old the last thing I wanted to do was spread strep so for the first time in almost 20 years, I took an antibiotic. But I knew this was not the last I had heard from the strep throat. After my supporting the natural healing ability of my body for so long, it wasn't going to let*

23

me get by with suppressing the infection and letting an antibiotic do the work for my body.

I returned to NYC and about a week later the strep throat returned again. This time I used tea tree oil on the back of my throat and drank and gargled with apple cider vinegar and drank liquid chlorophyll. And this time it went away and didn't come back.

Normally I will add a drop of oil to a small amount of carrier oil like sweet almond oil or jojoba oil, especially in the case of infants and small children. When it's me, I will sometimes use the oils neat (undiluted). If you do use oils neat, some oils heat up on the skin which can cause discomfort even pain. If this happens, use a carrier oil to dissipate the essential oil, not water, on the skin. Water will intensify the oil, not dissipate it. In a case like this I've even used canola oil in a pinch.

Some people can have skin sensitivity and oils can cause a rash. If this happens, discontinue use.

Topical application can take the form of massage, reflexology, or site specific application. Generally though, skin sensitivity rarely if ever occurs when using oils on the feet (although be careful not to rub your eyes or face – your feet won't break out, but these areas may if you are sensitive).

If you are using oils as a preventative, I recommend either diffusing or using them in routine reflexology sessions. Additionally, you will find application specific information below for colds, coughs and sore throats.

Essential Oils to Support Health and Wellness:

Listed below are some of my favorite essential oils that have properties which are consider anti-microbial (kills or inhibits the growth of microorganisms), antiviral (combats viruses), anti-infection (combats infection) and antibacterial (combats bacteria). When using essential oils to create a preventative environment during cold and flu season you want to make use of the oils that will kill germs and keep your environment clear of viruses and bacteria. In both topical application and diffusing you can make a blend of oils that both smells pleasant and addresses your needs.

Basil, Sweet (Ocimum basilicum): Antiviral, anti-inflammatory, anti-infectious, decongestant.

Canadian Red Cedar (Thuja plicata): Antifungal, antibacterial, insect repellent.

Cistus (Cistus Ladanifer/Labadanum/Rock Rose): Anti-infectious, antiviral, antibacterial

Clove (Syzygium aromaticum): Antimicrobial, antiseptic, antibacterial

Eucalyptus (Eucalyptus globulus): Germicidal and disinfectant (for children six and up)

Geranium (Pelagronium graveolens): Antibacterial

Lemon (Citrus limon): Anti-infectious, disinfectant, antibacterial, antiseptic, antiviral.

Marjoram (Origanum majorana): Anti-infectious, antibacterial

Tea Tree Oil (Melaleuca Alterniforia): Anti-bacterial, anti-infectious, antifungal, antiviral, antiseptic

Neroli (Citrus aurantium): Anti-infectious, antibacterial

Peppermint (Menta piperita): Anti-infectious, antibacterial, antifungal

Ravemsara (Ravensara aromatica): Anti-infectious, antiviral, antibacterial, antimicrobial

Rosemary (Rosmarinus officinalis CT 1,8 cineol): Antifungal, antibacterial, antiseptic

Rosewood (Aniba rosaeodora): Anti-infectious, antibacterial, antiviral, antifungal

Thyme (Thymus vulgaris CT linalol): Highly antimicrobial, antifungal, antiviral

Tool #9: Raw Juices

Starting your day with raw juices is a great way to set the stage for a healthy day. Your body will readily absorb the powerful nutritional benefits of the vegetables and fruits you choose. And where kids are concerned, you can often get them to easily drink raw juices by getting them involved in the making process. They love to choose what to put into it and to help with the juicing itself.

It's important when juicing fruits and vegetables that your end result be pure juice – no pulp. The body's ability to readily absorb juice diminishes once pulp is introduced into the process. But if your juice is pure, it's nutrients can be absorbed into the system in any where from 10 – 20 minutes.

There are several different kinds of juicers. For citrus fruits a simple hand juicer will work (you need to strain off the pulp), but for vegetables and other fruits a centrifugal juicer is the most practical (both expense wise and outcome). I've had a Juiceman centrifugal juicer for almost 10 years now. At present time, I think you can get a centrifugal juicer for as low as $99.00. These are juicers for first time juicers and if your interest in juicing holds strong, a better juicer would be warranted. So it is up to you if you want to invest in something around $200 or start with something a little less costly. Of course another option, if you are fortunate to live in an area where you have a health store that creates fresh raw juices, is to buy a fresh combo juice usually for around $4 or $5 a glass (about the same cost as a cup of Starbucks coffee.)

Here is a helpful site that allows you to compare many of the juicers on the market – this link will land you at the centrifugal juicers but you can check out the other types as well. http://www.harvestessentials.com/ceju.html If you want to use raw vegetable and fruit juices to account for your daily five servings – on average a 4 oz glass of pure, juiced fruits or vegetables is equivalent to ½ cup of the raw fruit or vegetable.

Fruit and Vegetable Juices

Apple: (not bottled apple juice)
- Vitamins A and C
- Supports healthy digestion
- Has been shown to reduce wheezing when a glass of apple juice is consumed daily.

Orange (not from a carton)
- Immune support – one orange supplies 116.2% of daily value of Vitamin C. (fresh squeezed – pulp free)

Carrot
- Aids digestion
- Promotes healthy mucous membranes

Spinach
- Cleanses, reconstructs and regenerates the entire digestive tract
- Excellent for addressing constipation
- Source of Vitamins C and E

Make it yourself!

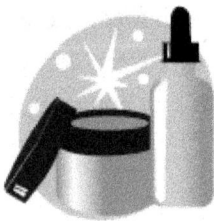

Health Recipe:
2 Apples
1 Carrot
Small piece of Ginger

Tool #10: Colloidal Silver Spray

There is a lot of misinformation out there about Colloidal Silver. When using a true Colloidal Silver there is no risk of argyria (turning blue). And it has been stated that it combats up to 640 known pathogens (including MRSA – the antibiotic resistant bacteria). I don't, however, recommend using it daily because in my experience it has the same potential to override the immune system just as the herb Echinacea can (I don't have facts on this – but it is what I see when I look clairvoyantly at Colloidal Silver in the body). I feel it's best to support and strengthen the immune system through diet, juices and reflexology. But Colloidal Silver is a great way to put the kibosh on a budding cold or other infection. I was using a spray that is 120 ppm (parts per million), but lately I've been using Soverign Silver which most health stores carry and it is 30 ppm. I use Colloidal Silver at the beginning of cold and flu season and as a preventative when strep is going around. For you or your kids - a few sprays in the mouth on the way to work or school and few on the return will help keep you fortified throughout the season.

Caution: There is a caution on the bottle regarding people who are sensitive to silver.

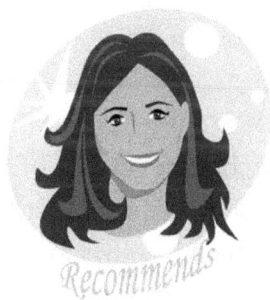

Recommends

Sovereign Silver – 30 ppm comes in a spray, a nasal spray and drops and is available at most health stores.

Total Silver Spray – 120 ppm (parts per million) available at

http://www.solutionsie.com/products/sie_total_silver.php

Tool # 11 Homeopathy

In the first edition of this book, I included Homeopathy as one of the 10 primary tools. I do love homeopathy and it does work really well, but it's not a preventative in the sense that it will boost your immune system and keep you healthy. It's more a preventative in the sense that if you are getting sick, it can stop whatever is developing before it becomes a full-blown cold or flu.

Homeopathy offers an interesting way to support the body's natural healing abilities. Used as a healing support for more than 200 years, it is based in the philosophy that small amounts of that which causes a condition can remedy it. For example, I get migraines, which can be caused by caffeine consumption. When I feel a migraine starting, I can often stop it in its tracks by drinking a small amount of Coca-Cola.

This approach is actually based in the philosophy of homeopathy, only with homeopathy you don't have the negative impact of the soda. Homeopathy is considered to be safe and almost side-effect free, unlike pharmaceuticals. Critics have claimed that positive results are "mind over matter." My response – is whether it enables the mind to trigger your natural healing ability or homeopathy truly works – what does it matter? I have used homeopathy and have used it with my son since he was born in 2004, it is a wonderful natural healing resource.

Traditional homeopaths work with one remedy at a time, but the process of identifying the specific conditions that lend to any given situation isn't always that easy when you are faced with a matter of urgency. When it comes to health and wellness, I prefer to use combination remedies. You'll find remedies for everything from coughs and colds, to respiratory problems like sinus and bronchitis to flu to constipation and diarrhea.

Homeopathy works on a less-is-more principle. You take the minimal dose necessary to evoke a healing response. If you choose to use homeopathy, this is a key place to let go of Western mentalities. More is not better. In fact, more may diminish your healing response. Follow the recommended dosages.

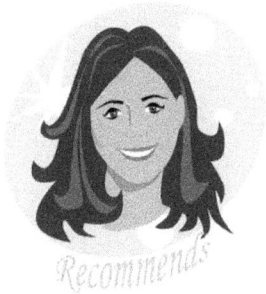

Although I could list specific homeopathic remedies, for the purpose of this book I'm going to refer you to two companies that offer combination liquid and pellet formulas. Personally I prefer mostly Newton Laboratories because their combination remedies are liquid based. Although I do have several of Washington Homeopathy's pellets and I can highly recommend them as well. Both company's remedies have helped my son Caidin with everything from teething to constipation.

Washington Homeopathy www.homeopathyworks.com	Newton Laboratories www.newtonlabs.net
Coughs and Colds # 16	OTC Complexes
Congested Head Colds # 81	Cold - Sinus
Cough # 17	Cough
Head Cold # 15	Flu
Influenza # 26	Kids Complexes (kids can also use the above complexes)
Influenzinum 08 – 09	Sniffles
Spongatos Cough Syrup	

Found in Your Local Health Store
I also recommend for coughs and congestion:
- Boericke & Tafel Cough Bronchial Syrup – available for adults and children (Health Stores and on-line) Comes in daytime and nighttime versions.
- Boiron: Chestal and Chestal Honey for adults and kids.

As well for Flu - Boiron Oscillococcinum which can be found at pharmacies, health stores even some grocery stores.

The Outside World? Out of Your Control?

Once we've addressed our internal world, we can shift the focus to our external world and how we move through the world every day. No matter how healthy we are on the inside, when cold and flu season hit and your co-workers are coughing on everything or your child's classmates forget to cover their nose and mouth when they sneeze, you want to be prepared to keep those germs away from you and your loved ones.

WASH YOUR HANDS!

"What kind of advice is that?" you say? In all honesty, washing your hands is one of the best defenses against viruses and bacteria. Every day we come into contact with countless germs and by simply making it a habit to wash your hands before and after preparing food, every time you come in the house and every time you use the bathroom (and change your child), you will greatly reduce your likelihood of catching cold or getting the flu. Germs are spread by hand to mouth contact and airborne (through a sneeze or cough). By washing your hands, you cut down on the number of germs you pick up and on the ones you can potentially spread.

If you have kids, remember the golden rule is "do as I do" not "do as I say." If you want them to wash their hands, let them see you washing yours!

Extra Support – Natural Hand Cleaner

Carry natural wipes or hand cleaner with you, so you can clean your hands after you touch door knobs, hand rails, shake hands, sneeze, cough, etc.

Below are two good recipes that you can place in a spray bottle – they contain essential oils that are antimicrobial, antiviral and antibacterial in nature. Remember to get pure therapeutic grade essentials – synthetic or poor quality oils will not offer the same healing support.

32

Make it yourself!

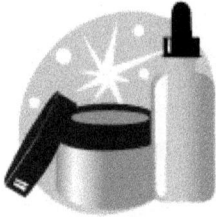

Makes 8 oz
Two 4 oz glass spray bottles
7 oz spring water
½ oz organic grape alcohol (190 proof)
10 drops Grapefruit Seed Extract
Therapeutic Grade Essential Oils:

More Floral
4 drops Lemon
2 drops Rosewood
1 drops Ravensara
1 drop Bay

More Earthy
2 drops Thyme
3 drops Geranium
2 drops Rosewood
2 drops Ravensara
1 drop Sweet Basil

The Dreaded Note From The School Nurse OR Bob is Sick as a Dog and Working Right Next to You!

If you have kids, whenever there is a case of something contagious at school, a note goes out saying "there was a case of strep" or "stomach virus" or "conjunctivitis" and to keep your child home if he or she experiences symptoms.

As soon as I get that note, I go into defense mode with my son's health and wellness, to help him stay healthy, rather than having to support him when he gets sick.

Remember the idea is to prevent first.

And what do *you* do when you go into work and there is good old "Bob" as sick as a dog? He's so committed to his job that he drags himself into work coughing and sneezing and in turn shares his germs with all his co-workers.

It doesn't matter what's going around; I begin regular reflexology treatments with anti-viral, anti-bacterial and anti-microbial essential oils, both in the morning before school or work and at night before bed.
(See Essential Oils and Reflexology for specific information.)

I step up natural juices and start Bee Propolis.

I also add Colloidal Silver spray. For a child, use before school and when he comes home. For you, carry it with you and use it three or four times a day.

And of course, wash your hands, wash your hands, wash your hands!

Condition Specific

No matter how much we try and no matter what we do, inevitably we're going to get sick at some point. It's just part of life. But hopefully, because you've been supporting yourself naturally, you won't get as sick and your recovery time will be far quicker.

There are many ways to address a single issue. Below you will find various natural suggestions that can be used when the noted conditions arise. You do not need to use all of them, in fact, it would probably be best to try one at a time so that you can understand how it works with your own body and what your response is.

If you are supporting your child, I also think it is best to try a remedy on yourself so that you know what your child will experience and can explain it to him as well. Remember, natural healing is a journey of getting to know what works with your own body.

Conjunctivitis/Pink-Eye

Colloidal Silver Spray:
If it's me and my eyes are feeling scratchy or I wake up with goop, I will just spritz my eyes with the Colloidal Silver spray. If it's my son, I'll place just a drop in the corner of his eye. Please note, the bottle does say to avoid the eyes. Do your own homework and research and decide if this is right for you or not.

Castor Oil
Castor Oil is a phenomenal natural healer. It acts as an anti-toxin. By placing castor oil in the eye before bedtime, it both soothes the eye and pulls the infection out. In the morning expect a lot of goop and continue with the castor oil until the eye is cleared up. Please note as well, the bottle does say to avoid the eyes. Do your own homework and research and decide if this is right for you or not.

Sore Throat/Strep Throat

Tea Tree Oil

At the first sign of a sore throat, dab the tonsils and adenoids (back side of the throat – where white would show up if it is strep) with tea tree oil. Saturate a cotton swab or place it on your finger and swipe the back of the throat. Repeat regularly.

Hydrogen Peroxide

Gargle with it and be sure to let it reach the back of your throat – just don't swallow it. Spit and rinse until your mouth is clear (if you swallow a tiny bit, that's ok, you just don't want to swallow it all.) This is my 'go-to'.

Apple Cider Vinegar/Hot Water/Lemon/Pinch of Cayenne/Honey

This is one of my most favorite home remedies for everything from sore throats to colds to coughs and even allergies.

Make it yourself!

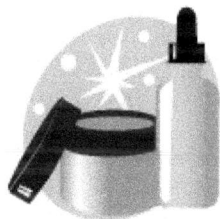

Heat up a cup of water
Add 1 – 3 tsps. of Apple Cider Vinegar
1/2 lemon squeezed
Pinch of Cayenne
1 – 3 tsps. of Raw Honey

Drink repeatedly throughout the day.

For kids – unless you have a spice lover, omit the cayenne – you can try adding a piece of ginger to generate some heat. (place the ginger in the cup and pour the hot water over it. Allow the ginger to steep in the hot water and then remove it. Then add the ACV, lemon and honey.
Caidin has been drinking this since he was four and he will drink ACV with honey. Our kids are all different, so find what works for yours.

Caution: There are warnings about honey and children under 1 year of age. The concern is that the honey contains botulism that the immature bowel cannot handle. Avoid giving honey to children under 12 months of age.

Oil Pulling

Oil Pulling is an Ayurvedic remedy that has been used for thousands of years.

By swishing Sesame Oil in the mouth it is thought to pull toxins out of the body. Another school of thought believes that the Essential Fatty Acids in the Sesame Oil are absorbed into the body and help fight infection and virus. Oil pulling is also great for any mouth problems of the gums or the teeth.

How to Oil Pull:

Use 30ml of Sesame Oil

Swish, chomp and gargle with the oil for 20 minutes.

DO NOT SWALLOW the oil. It is believed that the oil will contain bacteria pulled out of the body, so swallowing the oil is ill-advised.

Cold/Flu

See Sore Throat/Strep for Apple Cider Vinegar Drink

Homeopathic Remedy

For Flu: Boiron Oscillococcinum works well. It comes prepackaged for adults and kids and can be found in most pharmacies, health stores and even in grocery stores.

See Tool #8 for additional suggestions

Epsom Salt Bath

If you've ever worked with me on a health and wellness issue, you know how much I love the healing power of an Epsom Salt bath.

On the physical side, Epsom salt which is the mineral magnesium sulfate, has been found to help alleviate pain. Additionally, soaking in Epsom Salt helps to naturally pull toxins from the body, which speeds the healing process. When a cold or the flu is coming on, adding Epsom Salt to a before-bed bath, can often stop the virus in its track.

On an emotional level, I also find Epsom Salt baths to help soothe and calm emotions, again a result connected to the presence of the Magnesium. If you or your child is out-of-balance energetically, a bath with Epsom Salt will help you to settle and reconnect energetically.

According to The University of Maryland Medical Center 'Every organ in the body -- especially the heart, muscles, and kidneys -- needs the mineral magnesium.' 'Most important, it activates enzymes, contributes to energy production, and helps regulate calcium levels, as well as copper, zinc, potassium, vitamin D, and other important nutrients in the body.'

During a bath the body absorbs magnesium through the skin, contributing to the supporting effects of an Epsom salt bath.

Soaking in an Epsom Salt bath has the ability to pull toxins from the body while soothing aches and pains due to the natural magnesium content of Epsom Salt. I have stopped many colds from taking hold by taking an Epsom Salt bath before getting a good night's sleep.

What To Do

Epsom Salt Bath:
Make the water as hot as you can stand it.
Dissolve 1 cup of Epsom Salt in the water
Soak for 20 minutes.
Get out of the tub, dry off and get right into bed under warm covers. (It's important to do this as it will help you continue to release toxins throughout the night.)

For kids:
If you can keep your child from getting the salt water in their eyes, Epsom Salt baths have a comforting, soothing and calming effect on a child who is coming down with something, with the added benefit of helping to speed the road to recovery.

Place ¼ cup of Epsom Salt in a warm bath.
At the end of bath time, dry, dress in comfortable PJs and tuck them into bed.

Turmeric Milk

Turmeric is a powerful herb. It has many anecdotal healing properties with longstanding use in Aryuvedic medicine and Traditional Chinese Medicine. Westerners are catching on though and Turmeric is actually being explored through numerous studies including studies on its effectiveness as an anti-cancer agent.

I'm always perfectly fine with the 5000 year old history of use by the people of India and China. I find it curious that Westerners need to prove things before accepting them. In any event, that's an aside.

Turmeric is powerful anti-viral and antibacterial agent. It is also an anti-inflammatory and a carminative (prevents the formation of gas.)

When we have a cold our mucous linings swell. The Turmeric can help to reduce the inflammation and also decrease the mucous. With the flu, Turmeric helps to combat the virus through its anti-viral properties.

You can use Turmeric Milk as a preventive or once you feel a cold or the flu coming on. As a preventative, drink a cup a day. To combat an on-coming cold or flu; before bed take an Epsom salt bath and then drink a cup of Turmeric Milk when you get out of the tub, then get under the covers and go to bed. Drink another cup in the morning.

Kids can fair well with this drink, especially with the addition of honey (only use honey with children over 1 year of age.)

Make It Yourself
Directions:
1 Tablespoon of Turmeric
2 Cups of Almond Milk
Several Spoons of Raw Honey (to taste) – start with 2 tablespoons

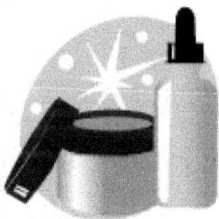

Heat all ingredients until hot, let cool to warm and drink.

Essential Oil

Diffusing Eucalyptus oil can help reduce fever, and ease the symptoms of cold and flu. You can also add a drop of Eucalyptus oil into a carrier oil and use in reflexology.

Caution: Eucalyptus oil is a powerful oil and should not be used with newborns, infants or toddlers and should be used with caution with children under the age of six.

Cough

Apple Cider Vinegar Drink
See Sore Throat/Strep for Apple Cider Vinegar Drink

Oil Pulling
See Sore Throat/Strep

Herbal Support
Elderberry is one of the most effective herbs in combating coughs.

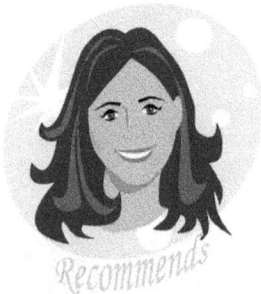

Recommends

I highly recommend Roots Remedies Immune Tonic. It is organic, sustainably harvest and made in small batches. http://www.rootsremedies.com/

You can also find Sambucus by Nature's Way in your health store.

For kids and adults:

There is a natural Berry Flavored version and a sugar free version
Berry Flavored: http://www.naturesway.com/?pid=15359
Sugar Free: http://www.naturesway.com/?pid=15331

Homeopathic Remedy

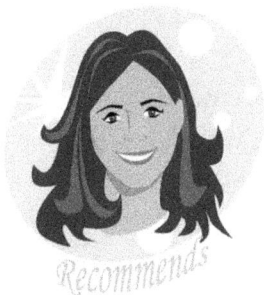

Recommends

- Boericke & Tafel Cough Bronchial Syrup – available for adults and children (Health Stores and on-line) Comes in daytime and nighttime versions.
- Boiron: Chestal and Chestal Honey for adults and kids.

My body has a pattern. If I get a head cold it inevitably turns into a hacking cough. What I have found is this: As soon as the head cold starts, I start taking Chestal until the head cold clears. I have successfully avoided it turning into a cough since I started this approach.

Also see Tool #8 for additional suggestions

Liquid Chlorophyll

Liquid Chlorophyll helps to build red blood cells and helps to remove toxins from the body. It naturally boosts the immune system also.

Drinking 1 tbsp in 8 oz of water one – three times a day when a cough is present will help alleviate the coughing.

Be sure to also drink several 8 oz glasses of water throughout the day to help flush the toxins from the body.

For kids:

If you can get them to drink it (I put it in a cup that can't be seen through with a straw and can often get Caidin to drink it – but as soon as he sees the "green" he's not interested):

½ -1 tsp of Liquid Chlorophyll in 8 oz of water

Diarrhea/Constipation

Constipation and diarrhea are at opposite ends of the spectrum but represent an imbalance in the healthy functioning of the bowel. If you experience either of these, it is essential to find balance in your elimination. I have found homeopathy to work wonders on these conditions.

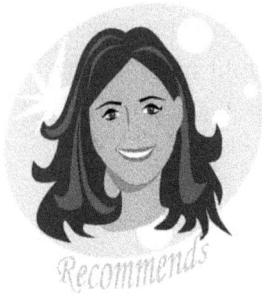
Recommends

For constipation and diarrhea I recommend the combination remedies available at both Newton Laboratories (liquids) and Washington Homeopathy (Pellets)

Constipation
Liquids -
Children ages 0 – 11:
https://www.newtonlabs.net/store/viewItem.asp?idProduct=106
Ages 12 and up -
https://www.newtonlabs.net/store/viewItem.asp?idProduct=243
Pellets:
http://www.homeopathyworks.com/jshop/product.php?xProd=265&xSec=109

Diarrhea:
Liquids –
Children ages 0 – 11:
https://www.newtonlabs.net/store/viewItem.asp?idProduct=146
Ages 12 and up:
https://www.newtonlabs.net/store/viewItem.asp?idProduct=396

Pellets -
http://www.homeopathyworks.com/jshop/product.php?xProd=261&xSec=109

Just In Case

Here's a quick check list of things to have on hand. Don't wait until it's 2 am and the stores are closed. Create a special holistic "go to" cabinet so you know where everything is. With natural healing, addressing a dis-ease state just as it is beginning will help you stop it before it takes hold, so you want to have your tools ready, should you need them.

- Raw Apple Cider Vinegar
- Raw Honey
- Bee Propolis
- Cayenne
- Liquid Chlorophyll
- Homeopathic remedies for flu, cough, diarrhea and constipation
- Elderberry Cough Syrup
- Homeopathic Cough Syrup
- Epsom Salt
- Tea Tree Oil (therapeutic grade)
- Castor Oil
- Colloidal Silver Spray
- Essential Oils of Choice
- Carrier Oil of Choice
- Sesame Oil

Wrapping It Up

I want to wrap up by restating what I said at the beginning. We are not alike and natural healing works with the individual. Where some of these tools may work wonders for you, others may not. Natural healing is a journey of getting to know yourself, empowering yourself to take responsibility for your own health and wellness and learning what supports your own health and wellness.

In some instances one approach may work where the next time something else may work. There is no quick fix, one pill, one-size-fits all in natural healing. Just as the tide ebbs and flow so does the body and depending on where your body is at in its ebb and flow, different support may be required for a seemingly similar condition.

As a parent, your knowingness and understanding of the body's ability to heal can extend to both supporting and empowering your child. I know that for Caidin, reflexology, when done right at the onset of a cold, will help him tremendously. And I know that I can put Epsom Salt in his bath and he knows better than to get it in his eyes. Just as each adult is different, each child is different. But for all of us, the more we are connected with our own bodies, the more empowered we become.

Use the information in the guide as a starting place and learn what works for you and your family. Let go of the belief that we need someone else to tell us how to support our bodies. Let go of the fear that your health and wellness is out of your control.

I hope that you will find this information helpful and supportive and that it will help keep you and yours stay healthy, happy and well.

Notes:

References

C. Leigh Broadhurst, Ph.D., Jack Challem Editor, *Basic Health Publications User's Guide to Propolis, Royal Jelly, Honey and Bee Pollen: Learn How to use "Bee Food" to Enhance Your Health and Immunity*. Basic Health Publications, Inc., 2005, Kindle Version, Loc 303.

Dr. John R. Christopher, (1996) *School of Natural Healing: The Reference Volume on Herbal Therapy for the Teacher,11th ed. Student or Practitioner,* Utah: Christopher Publictions

"Dietary Supplement Fact Sheet: Vitamin D", <u>Office of Dietary Supplements,</u> Dec. 11, 2008, National Institute of Health, July 10, 2009, (http://ods.od.nih.gov/factsheets/vitamind.asp#h3)

'FEELING PEAKY? YOU NEED MORE SUN! Good Health: As Research Shows Vitamin D Is Vital to Health, There's Only One Answer,' <u>The Daily Mail (London, England)</u> 3 Apr. 2007: 51, <u>Questia</u>, 1 Aug. 2009 <http://www.questia.com/PM.qst?a=o&d=5020097012>.

MF Holick. (2007) 'Vitamin D Deficiency'. *New England Journal of Medicine,* July 2007

Mark Pederson (1998), Nutritional Herbology, A Reference Guide to Herbs, Revised and Expanded Edition Wendell W. Whitman Company

Michael Pollan, (2008) *In Defense of Food, An Eater's Manefesto.* New York: Penguin Group

Janet Raloff, "The Antibiotic Vitamin: Deficiency in Vitamin D May Predispose People to Infection," <u>Science News</u> 11 Nov. 2006, <u>Questia</u>, 1 Aug. 2009 <http://www.questia.com/PM.qst?a=o&d=5028553219>.

Essential Oil Desk Reference, 2nd ed. (2002), Essential Science Publishing

William Sears M.D. and Martha Sears, R.N.,(1999) *The Family Nutrition Book: Everything You Need to Know About Feeding Your Children- From Birth Through Adolescence,* 6th ed., New York: Little Brown and Company

Dana Ullman, MPH, (1995) *The Consumer's Guide to Homeopath: The Definitive Resource for Understanding Homeopathy and Making It Work for You,* New York: The Putnam Publishing Group

N.W. Walker, (1970) *Fresh Vegetable and Fruit Juices. What's Your Body's Missing?* Tennessee: Norwalk Press

"What exactly are probiotics? What health benefits do they offer?" <u>Consumer Health,</u> Mayo Clinic, (http://www.mayoclinic.com/health/probiotics/AN00389)

About Christine Agro

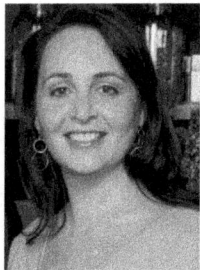

Christine Agro has Naturopathic and Master Herbalist Degrees from the School of Natural Medicine and she is an internationally recognized Clairvoyant, Metaphysical Expert, Spiritual Teacher and Natural Healer. Her work focuses on supporting women, families and children in all phases and stages of their lives.

Using her unique approach, Christine provides clients with a truly holistic overview of their health, wellness and well-being. She believes in supporting the body's natural ability to heal and in the power of natural remedies and support. Praised by grateful parents and celebrity clients across the globe for her intuitive and extraordinary gifts as a healer, she has been hailed as "magical", "transformational" and "inspiring."

Christine is the founder of The Conscious Living Guide™ (www.theconsciouslivingguide.com) TCLG is a membership site that offers additional insight, guidance and access to courses and workshops lead by Christine.

Visit www.christineagro.com for blog posts on parenting, pregnancy, conception, conscious living and animals; plus information on upcoming talks, events and courses.

Christine has been featured in *The New York Times* and in a Dutch documentary for *Metropolis TV*, interviewed on radio shows around the world, and quoted in health and consumer magazines and e-zines nationwide. She speaks to groups worldwide and does readings for individuals around the world.

Also by Christine Agro: 50 Ways to Live Life Consciously: 8 Tools and 42 Concepts to Help you Wake-Up and Live. (Haldi Press 2012)
Available at Amazon.com in Kindle and Paperback versions.

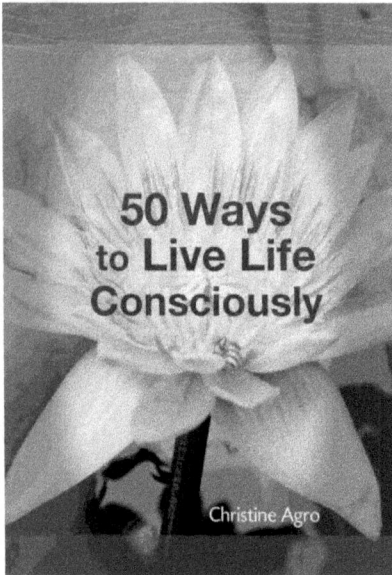

"Life is a journey. Spiritual evolution is a spiral. Living a conscious life puts you in the driver's seat of your own magnificently spiraling journey."

Christine Agro

We've been asleep at the wheel of our lives and the time is now to wake-up and start steering!

In this inspirational book, metaphysical expert Christine Agro shares 8 simple yet powerful tools, life changing insight into why we are here and how our lives work, as well as 42 concepts that encourage and support conscious living.

Have you ever wondered why certain relationships are so challenging, or just wished you could find greater balance and inner peace? Christine's information is simple and life changing. Once you read it, your view of life and the people you interact with will be positively changed forever.

Select Reviews

"You know you really love a book when you start reading and just have to take notes, and the notes turn into more like a book itself! " Black Diamond's Book Reviews

"Christine Agro brings to the reader in her book 50 Ways to Live Life Consciously an abundance of suggestions of ways to improve your life and enjoy it. " Rebecca Graf

"I loved the portion on "uncovering life lessons"... completely changed my understanding of the challenges & difficult relationships in my life. " TaraGreen

51

www.ingramcontent.com/pod-product-compliance
Lightning Source LLC
Chambersburg PA
CBHW071642050426
42443CB00026B/927